Table of Contents

Acknowledgments

Introduction

Chapter 1: About the Ebola Virus Disease

Chapter 2: What Causes Ebola?

Chapter 3: How Do People Become Infected with the Virus?

Chapter 4: Who Is Most at Risk?

Chapter 5: What Are Typical Signs and Symptoms of Infection?

Chapter 6: Complications

Chapter 7: How Is Ebola Diagnosed?

Chapter 8: When Should Someone Seek Medical Care?

Chapter 9: How Is Ebola Treated?

Chapter 10: Ways to Prevent Infection and Transmission

Chapter 11: What About Rumors That Some Foods Can Prevent or Treat the Infection?

Chapter 12: I Have Visited a Country Where the Ebola Virus Occurs. Should I Be Tested?

Chapter 13: Why Is It Unlikely That Ebola Will Spread in the United States?

Chapter 14: Should People Traveling To Africa Be Worried About The Outbreak?

Chapter 15: Are There Any Cases of People Contracting Ebola in the United States?

Chapter 16: The Ebola Zombie and Other Myths

Chapter 17: Food, Animals, and Ebola

Chapter 18: Chronology of Previous Ebola Virus Disease Outbreaks

Chapter 19: Ebola Trends Around the World

About the Author

References

Ebola

Demystify the Facts and Discover How to Keep Your Family Safe from the Ebola Outbreak

Dr. Timothy Moore

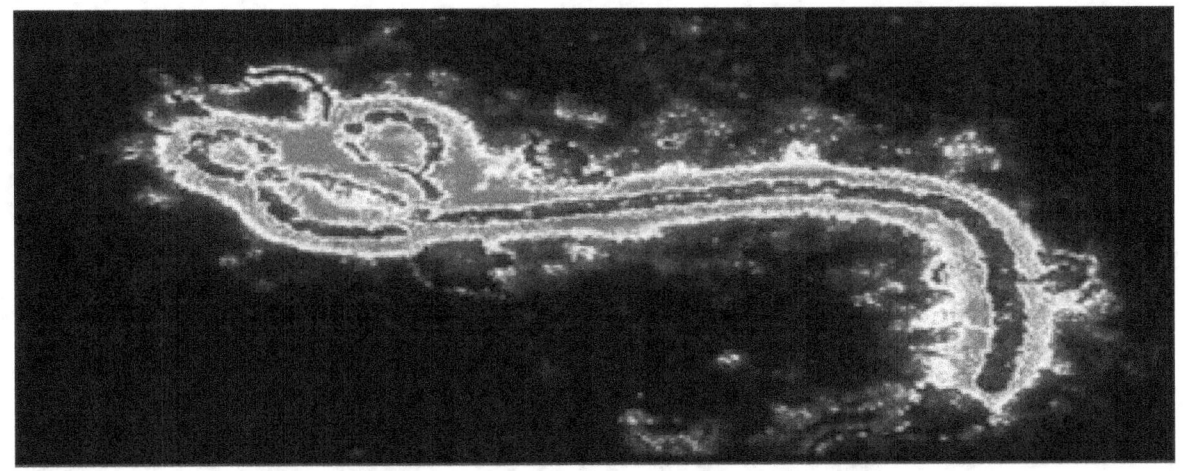

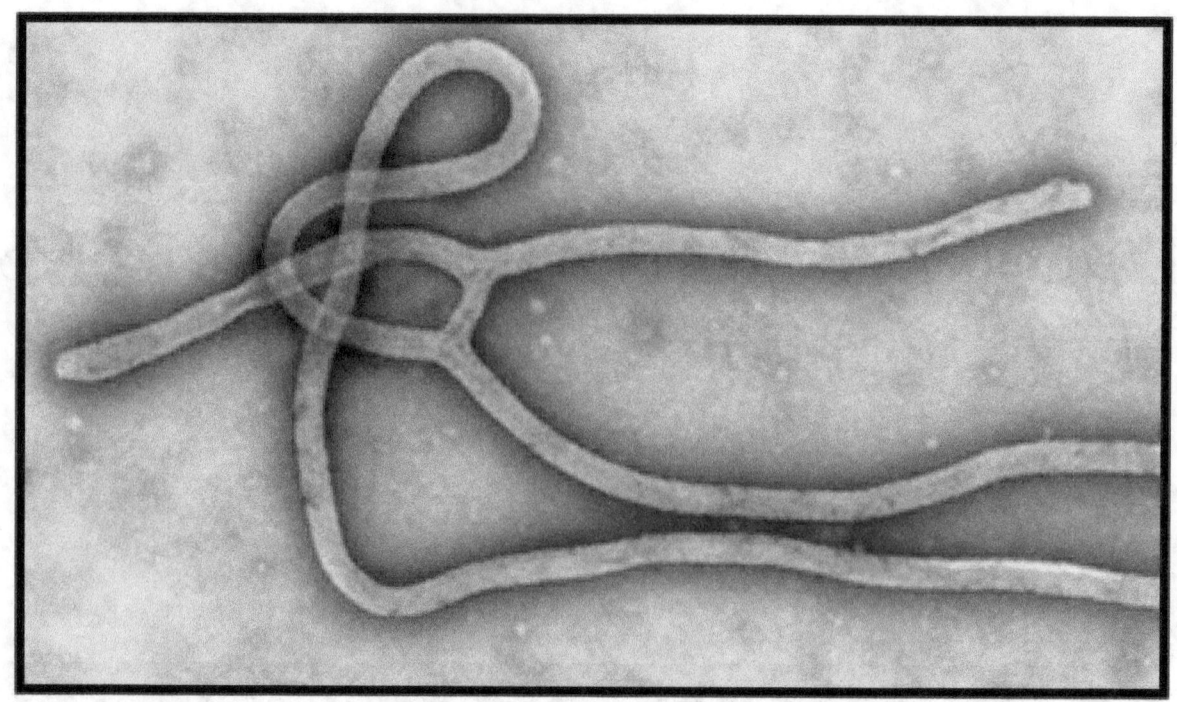

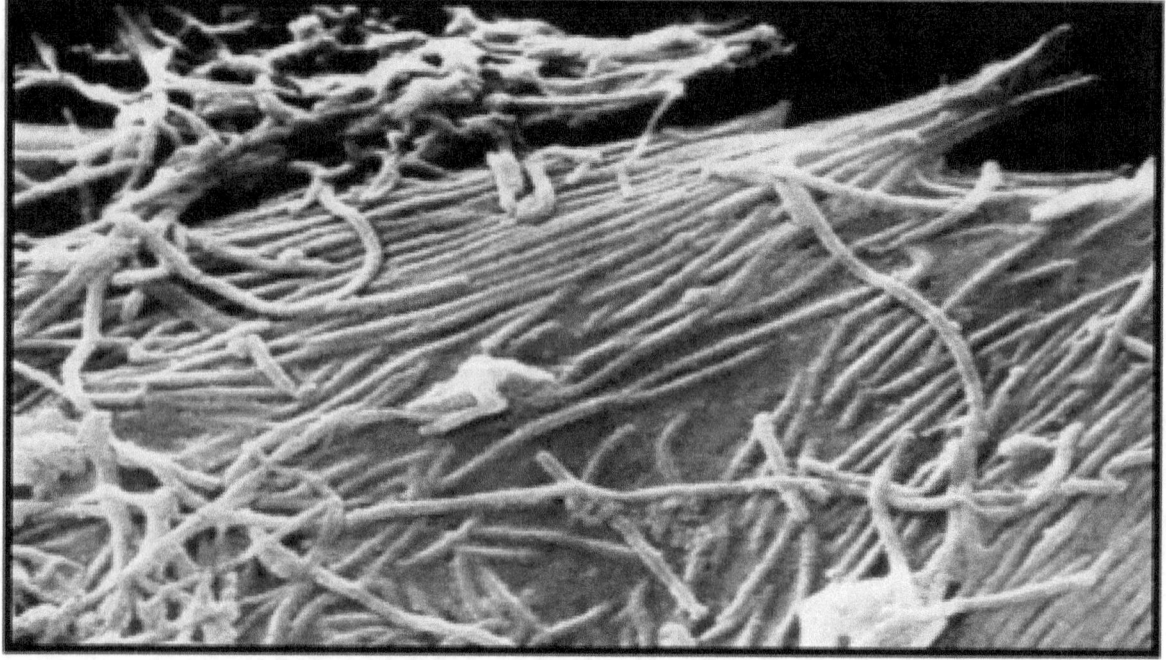

Ebola: Demystify the Facts and Discover How to Keep Your Family Safe from the Ebola Outbreak

Disclaimer

All material in this book is provided for your information only and may not be constructed as medical advice or instruction. No action or inaction should be taken based solely on the contents of this information. Instead, readers should consult appropriate health professionals on any matter relating to their health and wellbeing. The information and opinions expressed here are believed to be accurate based on the best judgment available to the author. Readers who fail to consult with appropriate health authorities assume the risk of any injuries. In addition, information and opinions expressed here do not necessarily reflect the views of every contributor to the book. The information in this book is presented for educational purposes only. It is not intended to be a substitute for the medical advice of your healthcare professional.

For more information about Ebola and for the latest Ebola updates, just scan the QR code above with a QR Code reader or scanner app from your smartphone.

Acknowledgments

Allow me to thank everyone who shares my life, our planet, our history, and our future. May I express my gratitude to my family, friends, and coworkers, especially those who contribute to and support the love of creation and development of this work. I would also like to extend my appreciation and wishes to you, the readers, who by your data, commitment to yourself, and your world, have enriched all of our lives.

Thank you.

Dr. Timothy Moore

Introduction

Ebola spreads and causes fear, but the question is: How do we contain this virus? We'll answer that in the chapters to follow.

Another important question is: How did Ebola land on American soil?

The chain of events we have to consider involve the actions and decisions of the United States government officials and the Center of Disease Control and Prevention (CDC). In the spring of 2014 Guinea, Liberia, and Sierra Leone began reporting to the U.S. that a surge of Ebola cases had begun to get out of control. By early summer, the African missionary workers reportedly contacted the U.S. health officials calling for an immediate response to the rapid spread of Ebola. Why did the CDC officials, both in the U.S. and in Africa, ignore this exploding epidemic of Ebola virus?

The U.S. did not ignore it completely, but it became a priority when an American missionary worker, Dr. Kenneth Bradley, was infected with Ebola. He was flown from Liberia to Atlanta, Georgia, for treatment of the virus with an experimental drug called ZMapp, and he fully recovered from the virus.

At the time of Dr. Bradley being treated, another missionary who contracted the disease was flown back to the U.S. and treated with ZMapp; a third was also infected and treated. As of this writing, there are three reported cases that were treated with this experimental drug; all patients improved and are virus free.

But why did the U.S. government officials fly infected patients to the United States, thereby risking the spread of infection on American hospital personnel, when they could have treated them with ZMapp in Liberia, Africa?

Also why did the CDC and prevention supposedly the world's leading infection control agency, fail to immediately assist Texas health officials when the first case of the Ebola virus was diagnosed on U.S. soil?

Last but not least, the important question is why are experimental Ebola vaccinations being fast-tracked into the human trials and promoted as the final solution, rather than to continue testing and production of the experimental ZMapp drug that has already saved the lives of several Ebola-infected Americans?

Barbara Loe Fisher is co-founder and president of the National Vaccine Information Center, a nonprofit charity dedicated to preventing vaccination injuries and death, providing public education, and defending the legal rights of everyone when making vaccinating choices. In the chain of events that occurred, Barbara summarized that there appears to be orchestrated failures permitting the disease to easily spread beyond borders, while still allowing government officials to fall back on excuses and possible deniability.

A logical conclusion is that some people in the industry,

government, and the World Health Organization (WHO) did not want the Ebola outbreak to be just confined to several nations in Africa because that would fail to create a lucrative global market for mandated use of a fast-track Ebola vaccination by every one of the 7 billion human beings living on this planet. Mrs. Fisher states, "Will there be an Ebola outbreak in America? Ask the CDC, the WHO, the DOD, the NIH, and Congress."

Chapter 1: About the Ebola Virus Disease

Ebola Virus Disease is a serious, usually fatal, disease for which there are no licensed treatments or vaccines. The experimental drug Zmapp seems to be the only thing giving people hope while ongoing trials aim to discover a cure for this disease. But for people living in countries outside Africa, Ebola continues to be a very low threat.

The current outbreak of the Ebola virus mainly affects three countries in West Africa: Guinea, Liberia, and Sierra Leone. Around 8,300 cases and more than 4,000 deaths have been reported across these countries by the World Health Organization in 2014. This is the largest known outbreak of Ebola.

Ebola virus disease (EVD), formerly known as Ebola hemorrhagic fever, is described by the World Health Organization (WHO) as "a severe, often fatal illness in humans." It first appeared in 1976 in two simultaneous outbreaks—one in Nzara, Sudan; and one in Yambuku, in the Democratic Republic of Congo. It is mainly found in tropical Central and West Africa, and can have a 90 percent mortality rate, although it is now at about 60 percent.

Infections with Ebola virus are characterized by immune suppression and a severe inflammatory response that damages vascular, coagulation, and immune systems, subsequently resulting in bleeding, multi-organ failure, and shock. Human-to-human transmission can lead to outbreaks, which are often initiated by a single introduction of the Ebola virus to a reservoir in nature, such as a lake or river, or from direct contact with an infected person.

The Ebola virus belongs to the viral family *Filoviridae*. Scientists also call it Filovirus. These virus types cause hemorrhagic fever or profuse bleeding inside and outside the body, accompanied by a very high fever.

The Ebola virus likely originated in African fruit bats. In 1976 and again in 1979, men working in a cotton factory in Sudan contracted Ebola. Fruit bats were found in the roof of the building both times and the bats are carriers of the virus, which can be spread through contact with bat droppings. The virus is known as a "zoonotic" virus because it's transmitted to humans from animals. Humans can also transfer the virus to each other.

To get more information, text your name and email to 1-(469)-530-0022

Chapter 2: What Causes Ebola?

As stated earlier, some animals are carriers of the disease, often after being infected by a bite from a bat. Animals known to transmit the virus include:

- Chimpanzees

- Forest antelopes

- Gorillas

- Monkeys

- Porcupines

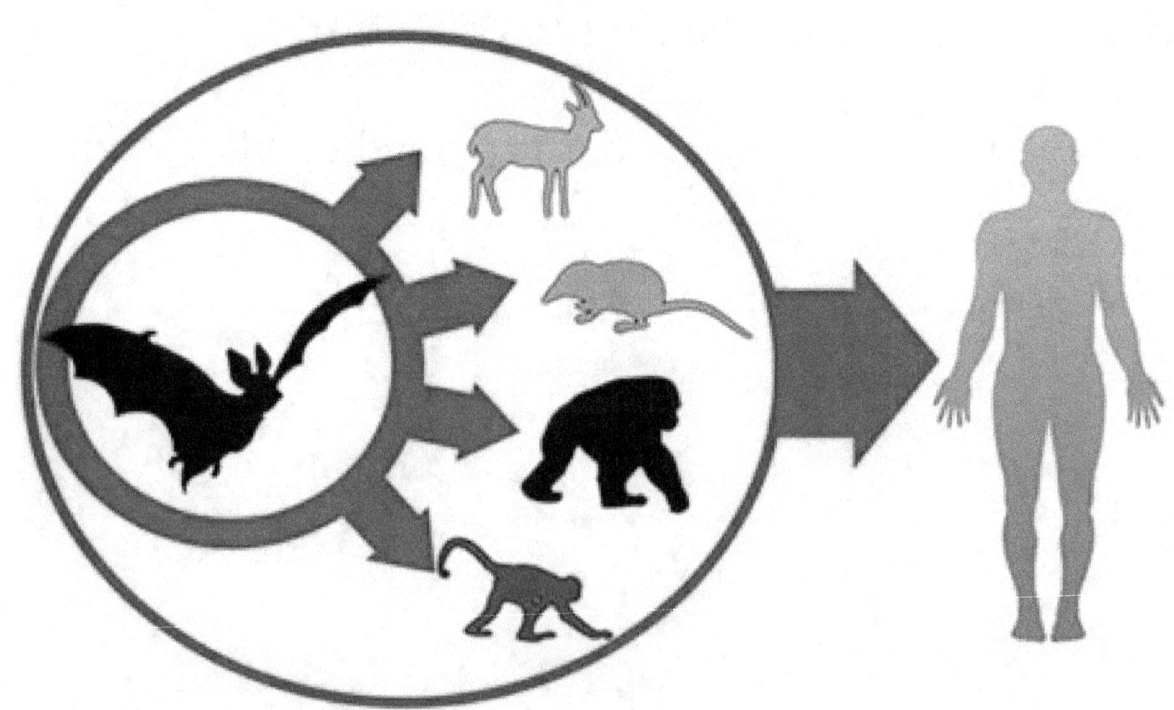

Since people may handle these infected animals, the virus can be transmitted via the animal's blood and body fluids. There is no evidence that the virus can be transferred by eating cooked meat.

Humans can also transfer the virus to each other through touch and from being in close proximity to an infected person. Once people become infected with Ebola, they can transmit it to others if people come in contact with their:

- Breast milk

- Feces

- Saliva

- Semen (According to the CDC, Ebola can live in the semen for as long as three months.)

- Sweat

- Urine

- Vomit

- Blood

These bodily fluids can all carry Ebola virus. As discussed in detail in the next chapter, people can get Ebola when they come in contact with these fluids via the eyes, nose, mouth, or broken skin. Healthcare workers are especially at risk for experiencing Ebola because they often deal with blood and bodily fluids.

Ebola can also be spread through being stuck with infected objects, such as needles, and with interactions with infected animals. To date, Ebola is only known to be transmitted from infected mammals and humans. Insects like mosquitoes are not linked with carrying Ebola.

Chapter 3: How Do People Become Infected with the Virus?

There are several ways to become infected with Ebola. Below are the most common.

(A) By coming in contact with body fluids:

Ebola has been detected in blood and many body fluids. Body fluids include saliva, mucus, vomit, feces, sweat, tears, breast milk, urine, and semen.

(B) Generally not by coughing or sneezing:

Unlike respiratory illnesses like measles or chickenpox, which can be transmitted by virus particles that remain suspended in the air after an infected person coughs or sneezes, Ebola is transmitted by direct contact with body fluids of a person who has symptoms o Ebola disease. Although coughing and sneezing are not common symptoms of Ebola, if a symptomatic patient with Ebola coughs o sneezes on someone, and saliva or mucus come into contact with that person's eyes, nose, or mouth, these fluids may transmit the disease.

(C) What does "direct contact" mean?

Direct contact means that body fluids (blood, saliva, mucus, semen, vomit, urine, or feces) from an infected person (alive or dead) have touched someone's eyes, nose, or mouth, or an open cut, wound, or abrasion.

(D) How long does Ebola live outside the body?

Ebola is killed with hospital-grade disinfectants and household bleach (chlorine is needed to kill the virus). Ebola dried on surfaces such as doorknobs and countertops can survive for several hours; however, the virus in body fluids (such as blood) can survive up to several days at room temperature.

(E) Are patients who recover from Ebola immune for life? Can they get it again, either the same or a different strain?

Recovery from Ebola depends on good supportive clinical care and a patient's immune response. Available evidence shows that people who recover from Ebola infection develop antibodies that last for at least 10 years, possibly longer.

We don't know if people who recover are immune for life or if they can become infected with a different species of Ebola.

(F) If someone survives Ebola, can he or she still spread the virus?

Once someone recovers from Ebola, they can no longer spread the virus. However, Ebola virus has been found in semen for up to 3 months. Abstinence from sex (including oral sex) is recommended for at least 3 months. If abstinence is not possible, condoms may help prevent the spread of disease.

(G) Can Ebola be spread through mosquitoes?

There is no evidence that mosquitoes or other insects can transmit Ebola virus. Only mammals (for example, humans, bats, monkeys, and apes) have shown the ability to spread and become infected with Ebola virus.

Chapter 4: Who Is Most at Risk?

For most people, the risk of getting the Ebola virus is low. The risk increases if you:

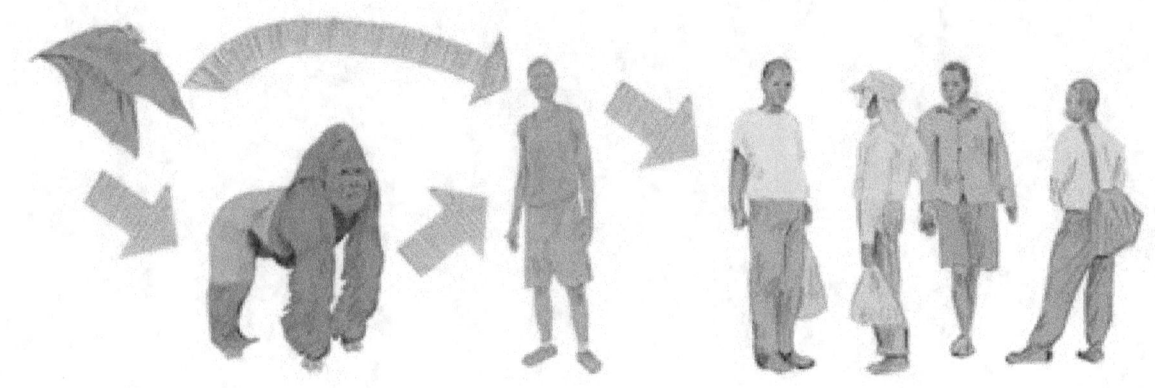

(A) Travel to Africa

You're at increased risk if you visit or work in areas where Ebola virus or Marburg virus outbreaks have occurred.

(B) Conduct animal research

People are more likely to contract the Ebola or Marburg viruses if they conduct animal research with monkeys imported from Africa or the Philippines.

(C) Provide medical or personal care

Family members are often infected as they care for sick relatives. Medical personnel also can be infected if they don't use protective gear, such as surgical masks and gloves.

(D) Prepare people for burial

The bodies of people who have died of Ebola or Marburg hemorrhagic fever are still contagious. Helping prepare these bodies for burial can increase your risk of developing the disease.

To get more information, text your name and email to 1-(469)-530-0022

Chapter 5: What Are Typical Signs and Symptoms of Infection?

Signs and symptoms typically begin abruptly within 5 to 10 days of infection with Ebola virus. Early signs and symptoms include:

- Fever

- Severe headache

- Joint and muscle aches

- Chills

- Weakness

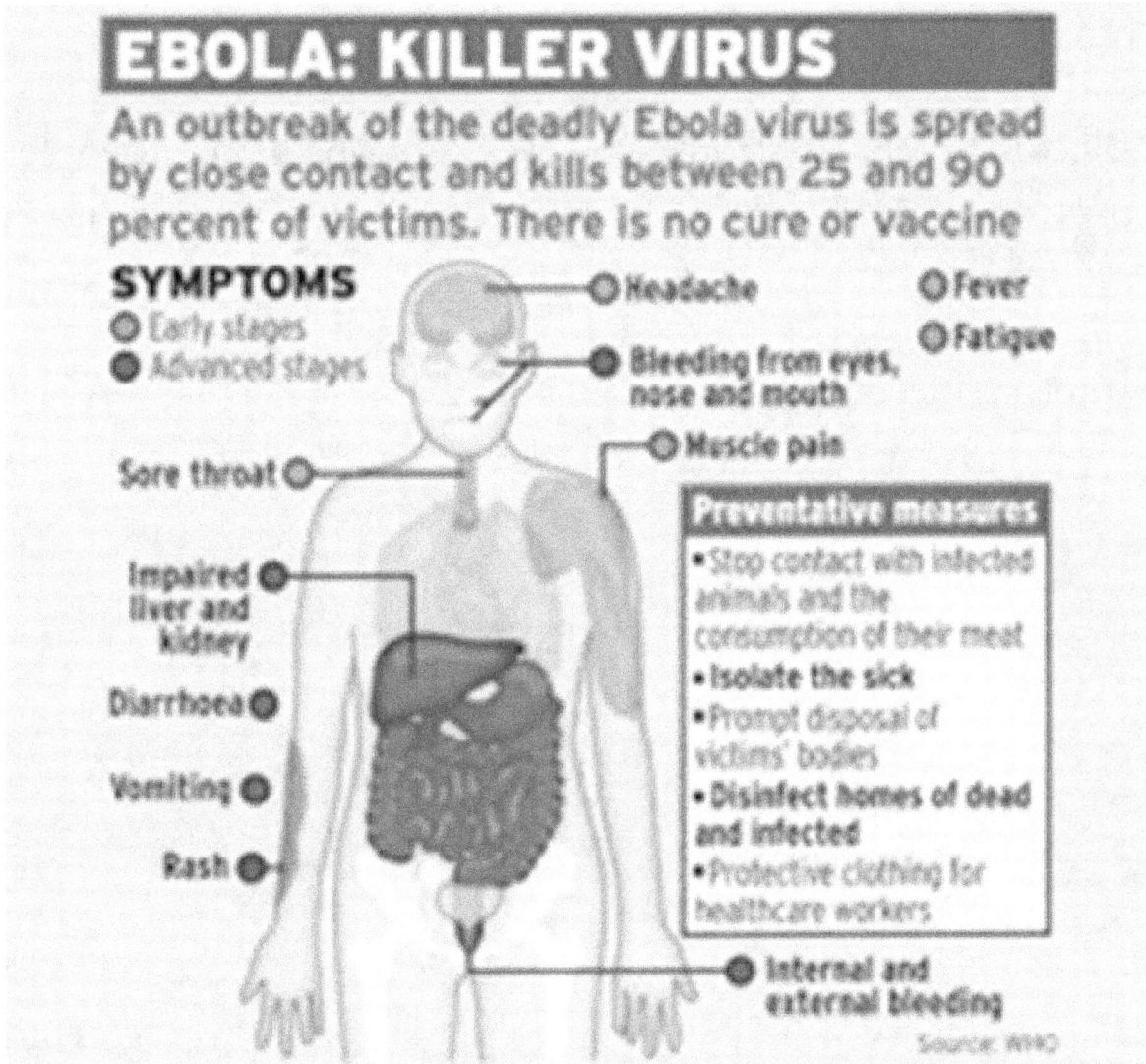

Over time, symptoms become increasingly severe and may include:

- Nausea and vomiting

- Red eyes

- Raised rash

- Chest pain and cough

- Stomach pain

- Severe weight loss

- Bleeding, usually from the eyes, and bruising (people near death may bleed from other orifices, such as ears, nose, and rectum).

- Internal bleeding

Chapter 6: Complications

Both Ebola and Marburg hemorrhagic fevers lead to death for a high percentage of people who are affected. As the illness progresses, it can cause:

- Multiple organ failure

- Severe bleeding

- Jaundice

- Delirium

- Seizures

- Coma

- Shock

One reason the viruses are so deadly is that they interfere with the immune system's ability to mount a defense. But scientists don't understand why some people recover from Ebola and Marburg and others don't.

For people who survive, recovery is slow. It may take months to regain weight and strength, and the virus may remain in the body for weeks. People may experience:

- Hair loss

- Sensory changes

- Liver inflammation (hepatitis)

- Weakness

- Fatigue

- Headaches

- Eye inflammation

- Testicular inflammation, which can cause sterility

To get more information, text your name and email to 1-(469)-530-0022

Chapter 7: How Is Ebola Diagnosed?

Diagnosing Ebola in a person who has been infected for only a few days is difficult, because the early symptoms, such as fever and flu, are nonspecific to Ebola infection and are seen often in patients with more commonly occurring diseases, such as malaria and typhoid fever.

However, if a person has the early symptoms of Ebola and has had contact with the blood or body fluids of a person sick with Ebola, contact with objects that have been contaminated with the blood or body fluids of a person sick with Ebola, or contact with infected animals, they should be isolated and public health professionals notified. Samples from the patient can then be collected and tested to confirm an infection.

Timeline of Infection Diagnostic Tests Available

Within a few days after symptoms begin diagnostic tests available are:

- Antigen-capture enzyme-linked immunosorbent assay (ELISA) testing

- Polymerase chain reaction (PCR)

- Virus isolation, IgM ELISA

Later in disease course or after recovery diagnostic tests available are:

- IgM and IgG antibodies

Retrospectively in deceased patients diagnostic tests available are:

- Immunohistochemistry testing

- PCR

- Virus isolation

Chapter 8: When Should Someone Seek Medical Care?

If a person has been in an area known to have Ebola virus disease or has come in contact with a person known or suspected to have Ebola and they begin to have symptoms, they should seek medical care immediately.

Any cases of persons who are suspected to have the disease should be reported to a local hospital or health care center without delay. Prompt medical care is essential in improving the rate of survival from the disease. It is also important to control the spread of the disease and infection control procedures need to be started immediately.

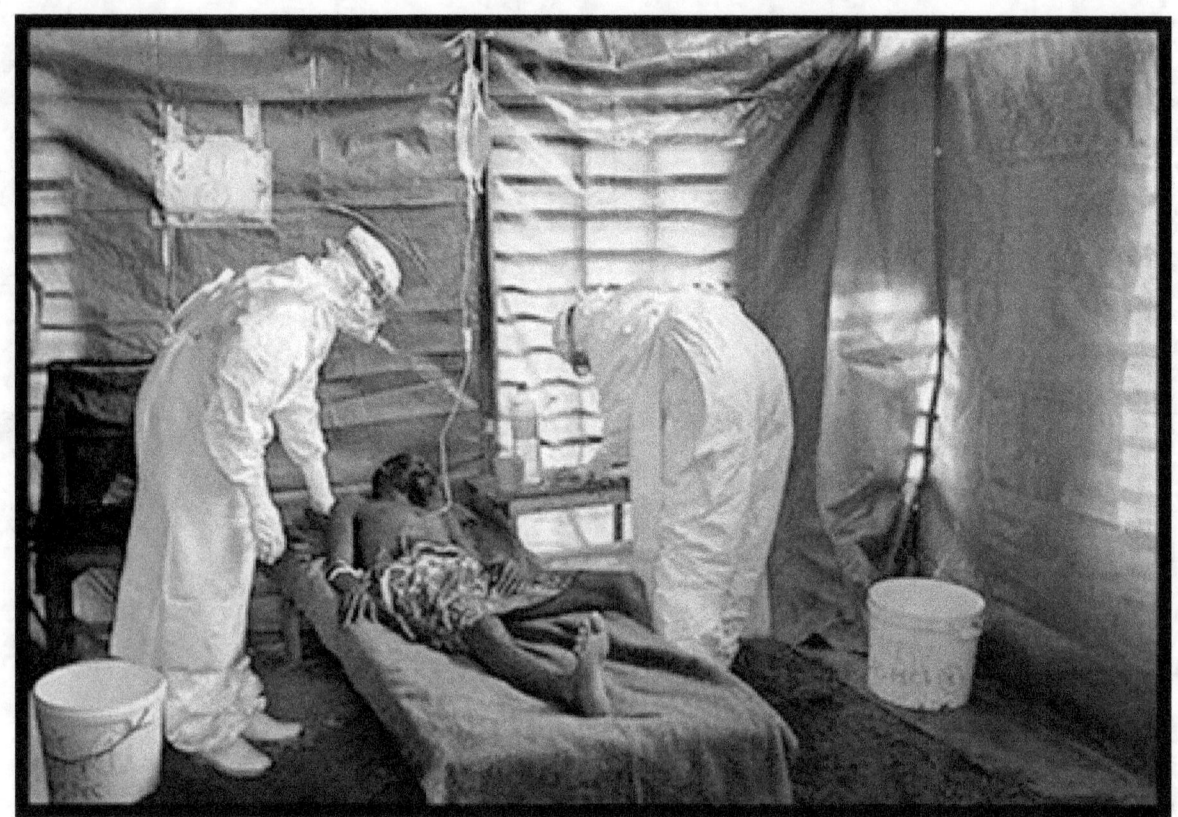

Chapter 9: How Is Ebola Treated?

The Ebola virus does not have a cure or vaccine at this time. Instead, measures are taken to keep the person as comfortable as possible. Supportive care measures include:

- Giving medications to maintain blood pressure

- Managing electrolyte balances

- Providing extra oxygen, if needed

- Providing intravenous fluids to prevent dehydration

- Treating co-existing infections (such as emphysema and cancer) and preventing other infections from occurring

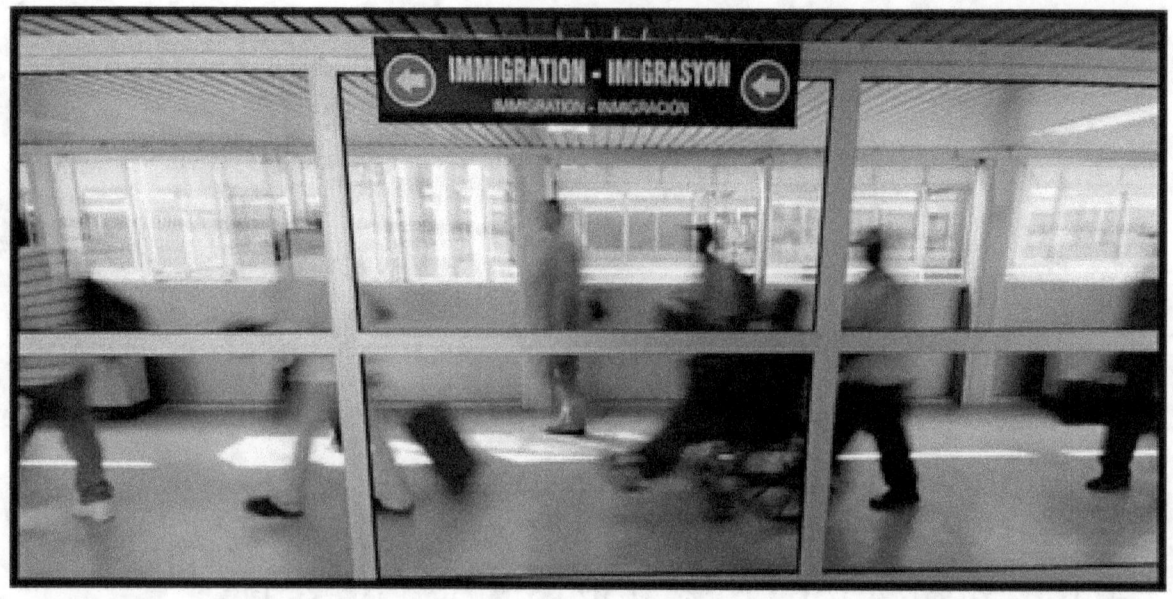

People's immune systems can respond differently to Ebola. While some may recover from the virus without complication, others can have residual effects like joint problems.

To help control further spread of the virus, people who are suspected or confirmed to have the disease should be isolated from other patients and treated by health workers using strict infection-control precautions.

Chapter 10: Ways to Prevent Infection and Transmission

While initial cases of Ebola virus disease are contracted by handling infected animals or carcasses, secondary cases occur by direct contact with the bodily fluids of an ill person, either through unsafe case management or unsafe burial practices. Casual contact with an infected person could potentially cause issues, but has not yet been proven.

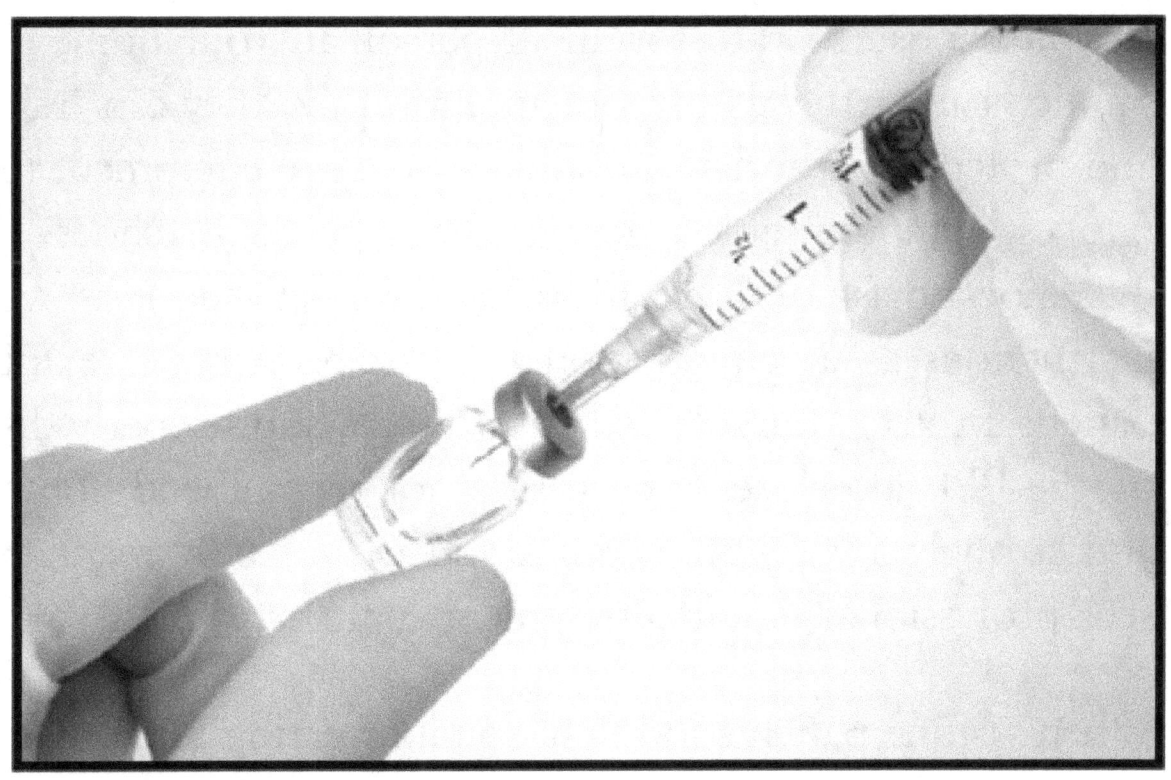

Several steps can be taken to help in preventing infection and limiting or stopping transmission, as published by the World Health Organization (WHO).

- Understand the nature of the disease, how it is transmitted and how to prevent it from spreading further.

- Listen to and follow directives issued by your country's respective Ministry of Health.

- If you suspect someone close to you or in your community of having Ebola virus disease, immediately encourage and support them in seeking appropriate medical treatment in a healthcare facility.

- If you choose to care for an ill person in your home, notify public health officials of your intentions so they can train you and provide appropriate personal protective equipment (PPE) (gloves, impermeable gown, boots/closed shoes with overshoes, mask and eye protection for splashes), as well as instructions as a reminder on how to properly care for the patient, protect yourself and your family, and properly dispose of the PPE after use. WHO does not recommend home care and strongly advises individuals and their family members to seek professional care in a treatment center.

- When visiting patients in the hospital or caring for someone at home, hand washing with soap and water is recommended after touching a patient, being in contact with their bodily fluids, or touching his/her surroundings.

- People who have died from Ebola should only be handled using appropriate protective equipment and should be buried immediately by public health professionals who are trained in safe burial procedures.

To get more information, text your name and email to <u>1-(469)-530-0022</u>

Chapter 11: What About Rumors That Some Foods Can Prevent or Treat the Infection?

The U.S. Food and Drug Administration is advising consumers to be aware of products sold online claiming to prevent or treat the Ebola virus. Since the outbreak of the Ebola virus in West Africa, the FDA has seen and received consumer complaints about a variety of products claiming to either prevent the Ebola virus or treat the infection.

There are currently no FDA-approved vaccines or drugs to prevent or treat Ebola. Although there are experimental Ebola vaccines and treatments under development, these investigational products are in the early stages of product development, have not yet been fully tested for safety or effectiveness, and the supply is very limited. There are no approved vaccines, drugs, or investigational products specifically for Ebola available for purchase on the Internet. By law, dietary supplements cannot claim to prevent or cure disease. WHO strongly recommends that people seek credible health advice about Ebola virus disease from their public health authority.

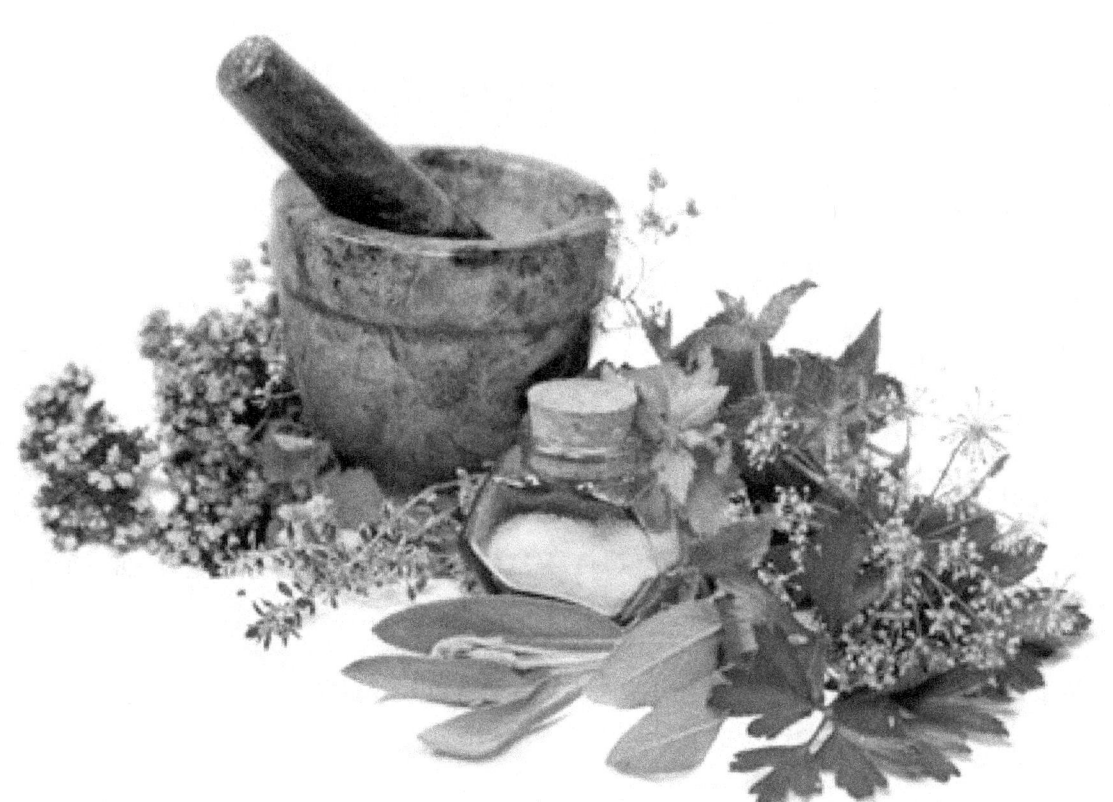

Chapter 12: I Have Visited a Country Where the Ebola Virus Occurs. Should I Be Tested?

For tourists or people traveling to Ebola endemic countries for business and who have had no direct contact with Ebola patients, the risk of infection with the Ebola virus is limited. Therefore, it is not recommended to perform standard Ebola testing on people without symptoms.

In case you have been in an Ebola endemic area, it is important to monitor your health in the three weeks after returning home. In case of illness, you are advised to seek medical advice from your doctor. However, symptoms such as fever, muscle aches, and headaches are also common in other diseases such as malaria or the flu. If your doctor thinks your symptoms might be related to Ebola it may be necessary to perform laboratory testing to determine whether you have contracted Ebola.

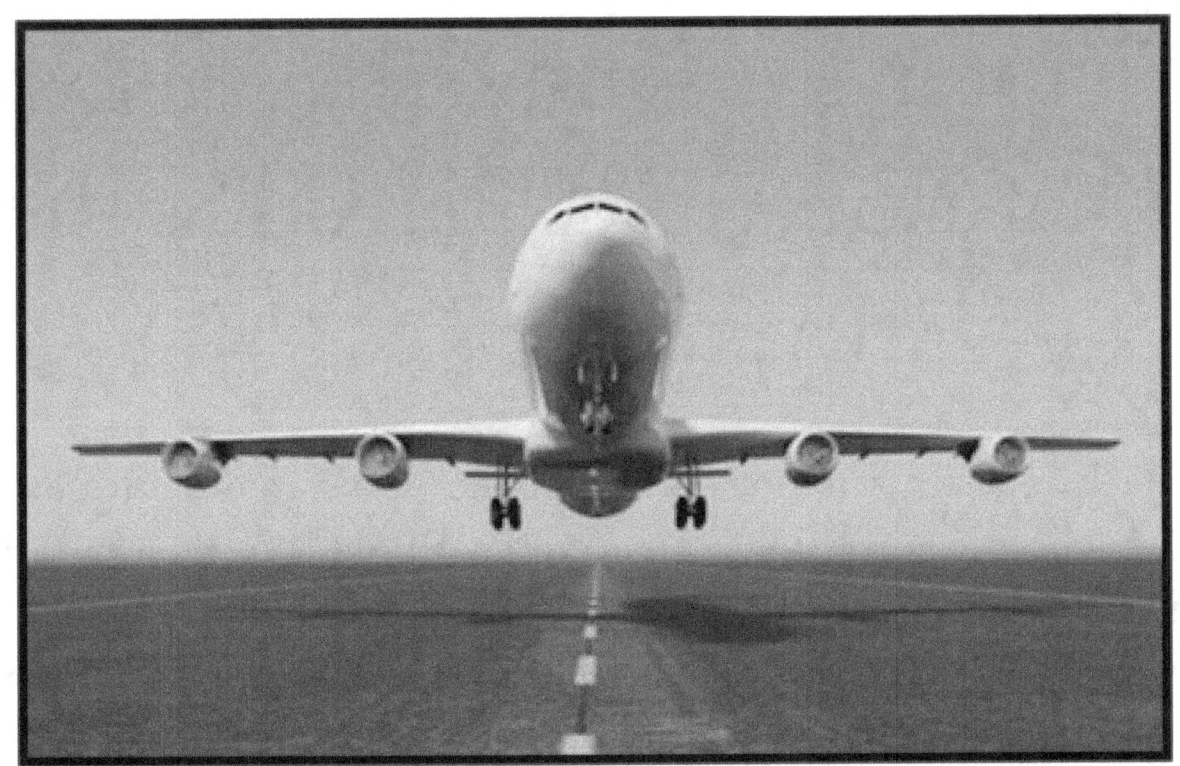

Chapter 13: Why Is It Unlikely That Ebola Will Spread in the United States?

The Ebola virus is not spread in the same way as influenza or other respiratory infections. To contract Ebola you must have been in direct contact with the bodily fluids of people who are already infected and have symptoms, or have touched objects contaminated with biological material containing the virus. The probability of being infected is therefore very low.

The United States health system is well prepared for cases where an infected person is transported to special hospitals for treatment. Healthcare professionals will use modern protective equipment and are trained to follow strict infectious disease control procedures. It is therefore extremely unlikely that the virus will spread further in the USA.

Cabin crews on planes are trained to react quickly if a passenger develops symptoms of Ebola infection during a flight to the USA from outbreak areas. They will adopt measures to limit the chance that other passengers will be infected, and will also notify the health authorities.

Chapter 14: Should People Traveling To Africa Be Worried About The Outbreak?

Ebola has been reported in multiple countries in West Africa. The United States Government has issued a Warning, Level 3 travel notice for United States citizens to avoid all nonessential travel to Guinea, Liberia, and Sierra Leone. A small number of cases were recently reported in Nigeria, but the virus does not appear to have been widely spread.

The CDC has downgraded the travel notice for Nigeria to a Watch, Level 1 because of the decreased risk of Ebola in Nigeria Travelers to Nigeria should practice usual precautions. CDC has also issued an Alert, Level 2 travel notice for the Democratic Republic of the Congo (DRC). A small number of Ebola cases have been reported in the DRC, though current information indicates that this outbreak is not related to the ongoing Ebola outbreak in West Africa.

The CDC currently does not recommend that travelers avoid visiting other African countries. Although a spread to other countries is possible, the CDC is working with the governments of affected countries to control the outbreak. Ebola is a very low risk for most travelers it is spread through direct contact with the blood or other body fluids of a sick person, so travelers can protec themselves by avoiding sick people, animals, and hospitals in West Africa where patients with Ebola are being treated.

Chapter 15: Are There Any Cases of People Contracting Ebola in the United States?

The government confirmed on September 30, 2014, the first travel-associated case of Ebola to be diagnosed in the United States The person traveled from West Africa to Dallas, Texas, and later sought medical care at Texas Health Presbyterian Hospital of Dallas after developing symptoms consistent with Ebola. The medical facility isolated the patient and sent specimens for testing and at a Texas laboratory that confirmed a positive test. The patient died of Ebola on October 8. Local public health officials have identified all close contacts of the person for further daily monitoring for 21 days after exposure. After 21 days of monitoring, if the person shows no symptoms of infection, they are virus-free.

Two healthcare workers (the second and third U.S. confirmed Ebola cases) who provided care for the initial patient have tested positive for Ebola. Both presented with low-grade fever and were isolated at Texas Presbyterian Hospital upon reporting symptoms. The CDC confirmed positive tests for Ebola for both healthcare workers. The second confirmed U.S. case was transferred and is now being treated in Atlanta at Emory University Hospital, and the third confirmed U.S. case is receiving treatment in Maryland at the National Institutes of Health.

The Health Ministry recognizes that even a single case of Ebola diagnosed in the United States raises concerns. Knowing the possibility exists anywhere, anytime, medical and public health professionals across the country have been preparing to respond. Public health officials in Texas and Ohio are taking precautions to identify people who have had close personal contact with the three confirmed domestic cases and healthcare professionals have been reminded to use meticulous infection control at all times.

To get more information, text your name and email to 1-(469)-530-0022

Chapter 16: The Ebola Zombie and Other Myths

A gruesome picture purporting to be that of a Liberian Ebola victim "risen from the dead" has gone viral online. The image is accompanied with the words: "For the first time in human history, confirmed footage of a man who scientists watched die from Ebola then only several hours later, regain life and rise from the dead." It then cites Bible passage Isaiah 26:19–20: "Your dead shall live, their bodies shall rise."

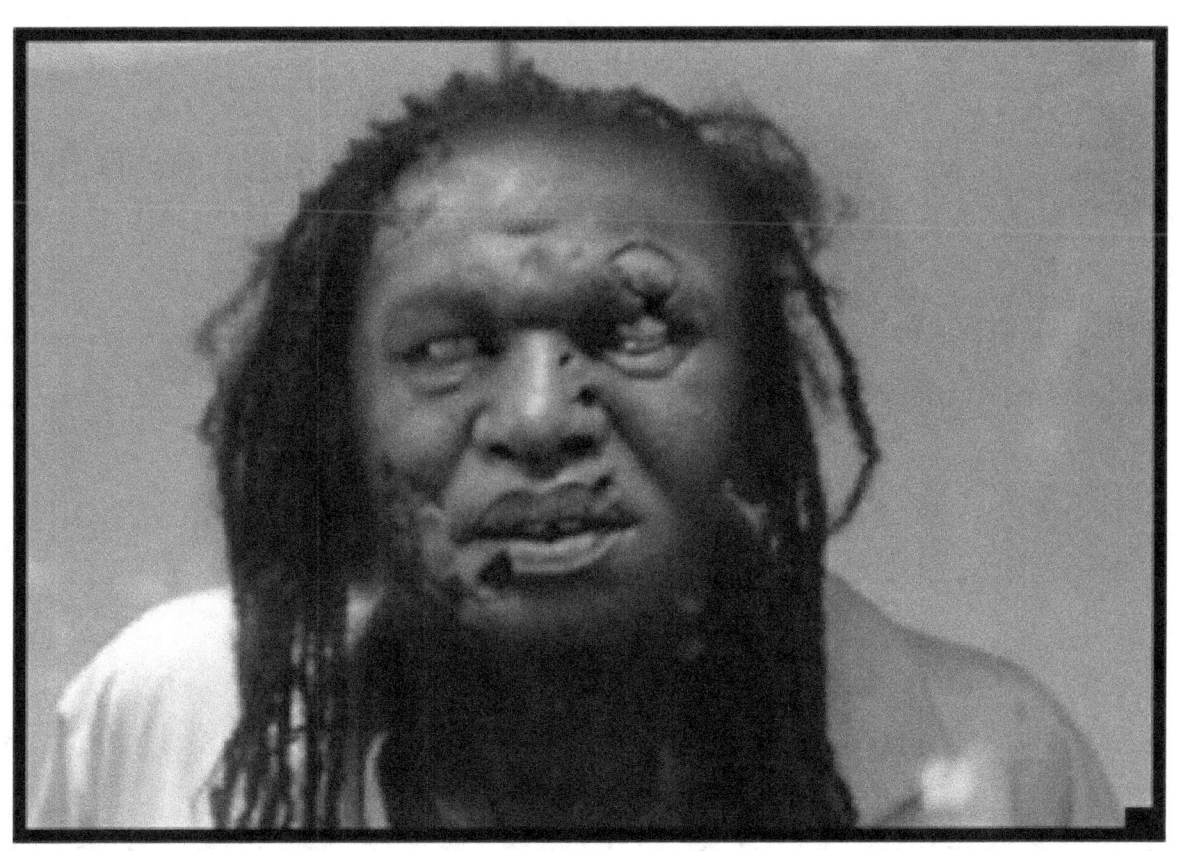

Warning of a possible zombie apocalypse, the article the image appears in goes on to claim the Liberian government has accused the USA of "creating Ebola as a bioweapon to be used in future wars." Needless to say, it's a fake. The image is hosted on the website "Big American News," home also to such juicy tales as "CONFIRMED: Obama is infecting Christians with Ebola to destroy Jesus and Start a New Age of Liberal Darkness" and "PROOF: Scientists Confess Hadron Collider is a Torture Device for God Particle." What's more, the image is said to actually be a photoshopped screenshot from the zombie movie *World War Z*.

Ebola Myths

1. If you go into a clinic and have Ebola, you'll be given an injection to speed up your death.

2. Routine blood tests and school vaccinations are a campaign to infect children with Ebola.

3. Ebola can be cured by home remedies, like a mixture of hot chocolate, coffee, milk, raw onions, and sugar.

4. Governments have fabricated the Ebola scare to deflect attention from scandals or depopulate rebellious provinces.

5. Health personnel and NGO staff are the ones spreading the disease.

6. Body parts are being harvested in the isolation units.

7. Ebola isn't real.

Chapter 17: Food, Animals, and Ebola

If food products are properly prepared and cooked, humans cannot become infected by consuming them. The Ebola virus is inactivated through cooking.

Basic hygiene measures can prevent infection in people in direct contact with infected animals or with raw meat and byproducts. These basic hygiene measures include regular hand washing and changing of clothes and boots before and after touching these animals and their products.

However, sick and diseased animals should never be consumed.

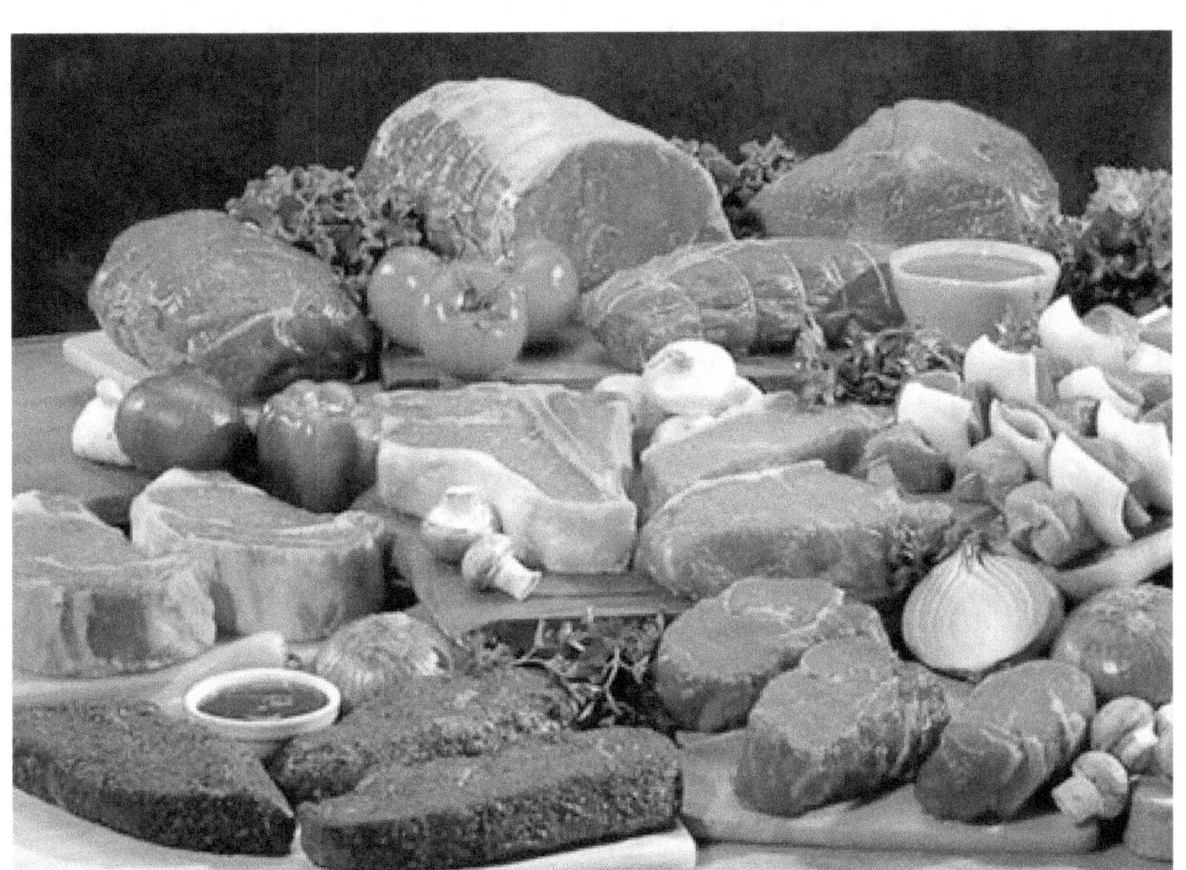

Chapter 18: Chronology of Previous Ebola Virus Disease Outbreaks

2012-Democratic Republic of Congo

Ebola Virus Species:: Bundibugyo

Cases: 57

Deaths:29

Fatality Rate: 51%

2012-Uganda

Ebola Virus Species: Sudan

Cases: 7

Deaths: 4

Fatality Rate: 57%

2012-Uganda

Ebola Virus Species: Sudan

Cases: 24

Deaths: 17

Fatality Rate: 71%

2011-Uganda

Ebola Virus Species: Sudan

Cases: 1

Deaths: 1

Fatality Rate: 100%

2008-Democratic Republic of Congo

Ebola Virus Species: Zaire

Cases: 32

Deaths: 14

Fatality Rate: 44%

2007-Uganda

Ebola Virus Species: Bundibugyo

Cases: 149

Deaths: 37

Fatality Rate: 25%

2007-Democratic Republic of Congo

Ebola Virus Species: Zaire

Cases: 264

Deaths: 187

Fatality Rate: 71%

2005-Congo

Ebola Virus Species: Zaire

Cases: 12

Deaths: 10

Fatality Rate: 83%

2004-Sudan

Ebola Virus Species: Sudan

Cases: 17

Deaths: 7

Fatality Rate: 41%

2003 (Nov-Dec)-Congo

Ebola Virus Species: Zaire

Cases: 35

Deaths: 29

Fatality Rate:83%

2003 (Jan-Apr)-Congo

Ebola Virus Species: Zaire

Cases: 143

Deaths:128

Fatality Rate: 90%

2001-2002-Congo

Ebola Virus Species: Zaire

Cases: 59

Deaths: 44

Fatality Rate: 75%

2001-2002-Gabon

Ebola Virus Species: Zaire

Cases: 65

Deaths:53

Fatality Rate: 82%

2000-Uganda-Sudan-425-224-53%-2000

Ebola Virus Species: Sudan

Cases: 425

Deaths: 224

Fatality Rate: 53%

1996-South Africa (ex-Gabon)

Ebola Virus Species: Zaire

Cases: 1

Deaths: 1

Fatality Rate: 100%

1996 (Jul-Dec)-Gabon

Ebola Virus Species: Zaire

Cases: 60

Deaths: 45

Fatality Rate: 75%

1996 (Jan-Apr)-Gabon-Zaire-31-21-68%-1996 (Jan-Apr)

Ebola Virus Species: Zaire

Cases: 31

Deaths: 21

Fatality Rate: 68%

1995-Democratic Republic of Congo

Ebola Virus Species: Zaire

Cases: 315

Deaths: 254

Fatality Rate: 81%

1994-Cote d'Ivoire

Ebola Virus Species: Taï Forest

Cases: 1

Deaths: 0

Fatality Rate: 0%

1994-Gabon

Ebola Virus Species: Zaire

Cases: 52

Deaths: 31

Fatality Rate: 60%

1979-Sudan

Ebola Virus Species: Sudan

Cases: 34

Deaths: 22

Fatality Rate: 65%

1977-Democratic Republic of Congo

Ebola Virus Species: Taï Forest

Cases: 1

Deaths: 1

Fatality Rate: 100%

1976-Sudan

Ebola Virus Species: Sudan

Cases: 284

Deaths:151

Fatality Rate: 53%

1976-Democratic Republic of Congo

Ebola Virus Species: Zaire

Cases: 318

Deaths:280

Fatality Rate: 88%

Source: WHO Statistics

Chapter 19: Ebola Trends Around the World

Nigeria reported it had Ebola on July 31, 2014, but there have been no new cases or deaths there since September 5, 2014. The densely populated city of Lagos (20 million people) has managed to escape the outbreak, which may be due to rigorous control measures.

The country is a hub for air travel around the world, so preventing a Nigerian Ebola outbreak is vital to reducing the risk that other countries will import a case. Other countries have only experienced small outbreaks.

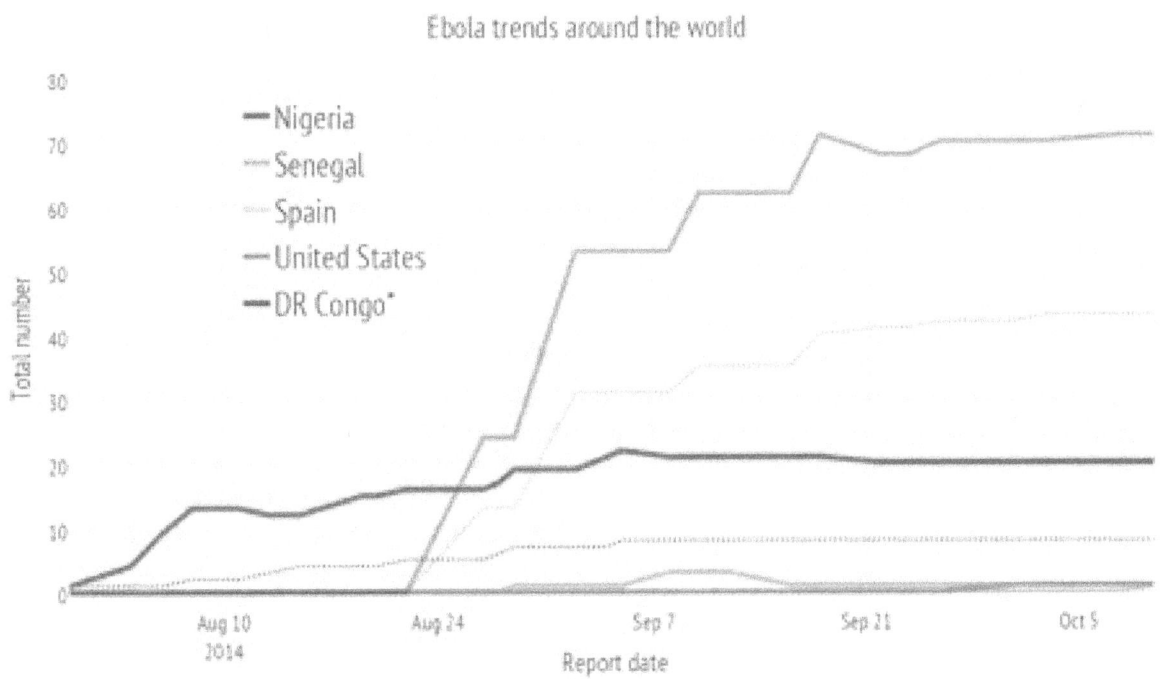

Ebola trends around the world

About the Author

Dr. Timothy Moore has spent more than two decades researching and practicing nutrition and progressive health care. He has received graduate degrees in both naturopathic medicine, and nutritional and religious science. In his role as an educator, Dr. Moore has conducted countless seminars, lectures, and educational programs across the United States and around the globe.

Because of Dr. Moore's progressive ideas on natural health compound with vast theological and practical scientific experiments, he has earned a reputation as a leading expert in the advanced field of nutrition and health care.

References

1. Li YH, Chen SP. "Evolutionary History Of Ebola Virus." *Epidemiol Infect.* 2013 Sep. 16:1-8.

2. Emond RT, Evans B, Bowen ET, Lloyd G. "A Case of Ebola Virus Infection." *Br Med J* 1977 Aug 27; 2(6086):541-4.

3. Roddy P., Howard N., Van Kerkhove MD, Lutwama J., Wamala J., Yoti Z., et al. "Clinical Manifestations and Case Management of Ebola Haemorrhagic Fever Caused by a Newly Identified Virus Strain," *Bundibugyo*, Uganda, 2007–2008. PLoS One. 2012; 7(12):e52986.

4. European Centre for Disease Prevention and Control. "ECDC Fact Sheet: Ebola and Marburg Fever [internet]." ECDC; 2014 [cited 2014 Mar 20]. Available from: http://www.ecdc.europa.eu/en/healthtopics/ebola_marburg_fevers

5. Bannister B. "Viral Haemorrhagic Fevers Imported into Non-Endemic Countries: Risk Assessment and Management." *Br Med Bull* 2010; 95:193-225.

6. World Health Organization. "Ebola Haemorrhagic Fever - Fact Sheet [internet]." WHO Media centre; 2012 [cited 2014 Mar 20]. Available from: http://www.who.int/mediacentre/factsheets/fs103/en/.

7. Martini G.A., Schmidt H.A. "Spermatogenic Transmission of the 'Marburg Virus'. (Causes of 'Marburg Simian Disease')". Klin

Wochenschr. 1968 Apr 1; 46(7):398-400.

8. Muyembe-Tamfum J.J., Mulangu S., Masumu J., Kayembe J.M., Kemp A., Paweska J.T. "Ebola Virus Outbreaks in Africa: Past and Present." Onderstepoort J Vet Res. 2012; 79(2):451.

9. Wood JL, Leach M, Waldman L, Macgregor H, Fooks AR, Jones KE, et al. A framework for the study of zoonotic disease emergence and its drivers: spillover of bat pathogens as a case study. Philos Trans R Soc Lond B Biol Sci. 2012 Oct 19; 367(1604):2881-92.

10. Hayman DT, Yu M, Crameri G, Wang LF, Suu-Ire R, Wood JL, et al. Ebola virus antibodies in fruit bats, Ghana, West Africa. Emerg Infect Dis. 2012 Jul; 18(7):1207-9.

11. Pourrut X, Delicat A, Rollin PE, Ksiazek TG, Gonzalez JP, Leroy EM. Spatial and temporal patterns of Zaire ebolavirus antibody prevalence in the possible reservoir bat species. J Infect Dis. 2007 Nov 15; 196 Suppl 2:S176-83.

12. Piercy TJ, Smither SJ, Steward JA, Eastaugh L, Lever MS. The survival of filoviruses in liquids, on solid substrates and in a dynamic aerosol. J Appl Microbiol. 2010 Nov; 109(5):1531-9.

13. Public Health Agency of Canada. Ebola virus. Pathogen Safety Data Sheet - Infectious substances [internet]. Public Health Agency of Canada.; 2010 [cited 2014 Mar 31]. Available from: http://www.phac-aspc.gc.ca/lab-bio/res/psds-ftss/ebola-eng.php..

14. Colebunders R, Borchert M. Ebola haemorrhagic fever--a review. J Infect. 2000 Jan; 40(1):16-20.

15. Dowell SF, Mukunu R, Ksiazek TG, Khan AS, Rollin PE, Peters CJ. Transmission of Ebola hemorrhagic fever: a study of risk factors in family members, Kikwit, Democratic Republic of the Congo, 1995. Commission de Lutte contre les Epidemies a Kikwit. J Infect Dis. 1999 Feb; 179 Suppl 1:S87-91.

16. Francesconi P, Yoti Z, Declich S, Onek PA, Fabiani M, Olango J, et al. Ebola hemorrhagic fever transmission and risk factors of contacts, Uganda. Emerg Infect Dis. 2003 Nov; 9(11):1430-7.

17. Raabea VN, Borcherta M. Infection control during filoviral hemorrhagic Fever outbreaks. J Glob Infect Dis. 2012 Jan; 4(1):69-74.

18. Ftika L, Maltezou HC. Viral haemorrhagic fevers in healthcare settings. J Hosp Infect. 2013 Mar; 83(3): 185-92.

19. Formenty P, Hatz C, Le Guenno B, Stoll A, Rogenmoser P, Widmer A. Human infection due to Ebola virus, subtype Cote d'Ivoire: clinical and biologic presentation. J Infect Dis. 1999 Feb; 179 Suppl 1:S48-53.

20. World Health Organization. Ebola haemorrhagic fever - Global Alert and Response (GAR). [internet]. 2014 [cited 2014 Mar 22]. Available from: http://www.who.int/csr/disease/ebola/en/.

21. Feldmann H, Jones S, Klenk HD, Schnittler HJ. Ebola virus: from discovery to vaccine. Nat Rev Immunol. 2003 Aug; 3(8):677-85.

22. Marzi A, Feldmann H. Ebola virus vaccines: an overview of current approaches. Expert Rev Vaccines. 2014 Apr; 13(4):521-31.

23. Saphire EO. An update on the use of antibodies against the filoviruses. Immunotherapy. 2013 Nov; 5(11):1221-33.

24. National Reference Center for Viral Hemorrhagic Fevers, Unit of Biology of Emerging Viral Infection. Institut Pasteur/INSERM. BSL4 Laboratory (Sylvain Baize and Delphine Pannetier). Ebola virus disease – West Africa: Guinea, Zaire Ebola virus suspected. [internet]. Promed; 2014 [cited 2014 Mar 23]. Available from: http://www.promedmail.org/direct.php?id=2349865.

25. Reuters. Guinea confirms fever is Ebola, has killed up to 59 [internet]. 2014 [22 March 20124]. Available from: http://in.reuters.com/article/2014/03/22/us-guinea-ebola-idINBREA2L0MI20140322.

26. Agence France Presse. Guinea confirms Ebola as source of deadly epidemic [internet]. 2014 [cited 2014 Mar 22]. Available from: http://www.google.com/hostednews/afp/article/ALeqM5jJ28KtrT docId=d1ac2db4-7d42-45d8-9130-daf4f0bd1f4c&hl=en.

27. World Health Organization, Regional Office for Africa. Ebola virus disease, West Africa (Situation as of 1 April 2014) [internet]. 2014 [cited 2014 Apr 1]. Available from: http://www.afro.who.int/en/clusters-a-programmes/dpc/epidemic-a-pandemic-alert-and-response/outbreak-news/4074-ebola-virus-disease-west-africa-2-april-2014.html.

28. World Health Organization, Regional Office for Africa. Ebola virus disease, West Africa (Situation as of 7 April 2014) [internet]. 2014 [cited 2014 Apr 7]. Available from:

http://www.afro.who.int/en/clusters-a-programmes/dpc/epidemic-a-pandemic-alert-and-response/outbreak-news/4087-ebola-virus-disease-west-africa-7-april-2014.html.

29. Republic of Liberia, Ministry of Health and Social Welfare. Press release [internet]. 2014 [cited 2014 Mar 31]. Available from: http://www.mohsw.gov.lr/documents/march%2031,%202014.pdf..

30. World Health Organization, Regional Office for Africa. Dashboard – Ebola Virus Disease in West Africa (7 April 2014) [internet]. 2014 [cited 2014 Apr 7]. Available from: http://www.afro.who.int/en/clusters-a-programmes/dpc/epidemic-a-pandemic-alert-and-response/outbreak-news/4089-dashboard-ebola-virus-disease-in-west-africa-07-april-2014.html.

31. Bureau de Presse de la Présidence. Epidémie de fièvre virale hémorragique en Guinée : déclaration du ministère de la sante [internet]. 2014 [cited 2014 Mar 21]. Available from: http://www.lexpressguinee.com/fichiers/blog16-999.php?pseudo=rub2&code=calb4122&langue=fr.

32. BBC News Africa. Guinea Ebola outbreak: Bat-eating banned to curb virus [internet]. 2014 [cited 2014 Apr 1]. Available from: http://www.bbc.com/news/world-africa-26735118#?utm_source=twitterfeed&utm_medium=twitter.

33. The French Ministry of Foreign Affairs. Conseils aux voyageurs (Travel Advice) [internet]. 2014 [cited 2014 Mar 22]. Available from: http://www.diplomatie.gouv.fr/fr/conseils-aux-voyageurs/conseils-par-pays/guinee-12255/.

34. Ambassade de France en Guinée. Message de sécurité : fièvre Ebola en Guinée Forestière [internet]. 2014 [cited 2014 Mar 23]. Available from: http://www.ambafrance-gn.org/Message-de-securite-fievre.

35. Ministère des Affaires sociales et de la Santé Fièvre hémorragique à virus Ebola [internet]. 2014 [cited 2014 Mar 26]. Available from: http://www.sante.gouv.fr/fievre-hemorragique-a-virus-ebola.html.

36. Reuters. Senegal shuts land border with Guinea to prevent Ebola spreading [internet]. 2014 [cited 2014 Mar 29]. Available from: http://www.reuters.com/article/2014/03/29/us-guinea-ebola-idUSBREA2S0JA20140329.

37. Public Health Agency of Canada. Travel Health Notice - Ebola Outbreak in Guinea. [internet]. 2014 [cited 2014 Mar 26]. Available from: http://www.phac-aspc.gc.ca/tmp-pmv/notices-avis/notices-avis-eng.php?id=125.

38. Boiro I, Lomonossov NN, Sotsinski VA, Constantinov OK, Tkachenko EA, Inapogui AP, et al. [Clinico-epidemiologic and laboratory research on hemorrhagic fevers in Guinea]. Bull Soc Pathol Exot Filiales. 1987; 80(4):607-12.

39. Conakry Airport [internet]. 2014 [cited 2014 Mar 22]. Available from: http://www.kinkaa.fr/aeroports/Conakry_CKY.

40. European Centre for Disease Prevention and Control. Risk assessment guidelines for diseases transmitted on aircraft. 2nd ed. Stockholm: ECDC; 2010. Available from:

http://ecdc.europa.eu/en/publications/publications/1012_gui_ragi

41. World Health Organization. A Guide for Shippers of Infectious Substances, 2013 [internet]. 2014 [cited 2014 Mar 22]. Available from: http://www.who.int/ihr/infectious_substances/en/.

42. Chepurnov AA, Chuev Iu P, P'Iankov O V, Efimova IV. "The Effect of Some Physical and Chemical Factors on Inactivation of the Ebola Virus." Vopr Virusol. 1995 Mar-Apr; 40(2):74-6.

For more information about Ebola and for the latest Ebola updates, just scan the QR code above with a QR Code reader or scanner app from your smartphone.